SHAK THERAPY

Regain speech and limb movement after a stroke or head trauma accident, far quicker than most conventional methods

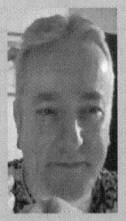

JOHN W GREEN

Shak 'stroke' Therapy

Speed up your recovery time!

Many stroke survivors has been introduced to a very unique therapy developed by John W Green in 1986; that has some cases miraculously fully healed Survivors who thought they would never again regain their normal bodily reflex/ cognitive functions; yet! Have suddenly regained perfect speech, moved limbs at will, got up and walked without the aid of a walking stick.

Read how this have been made possible and how you can learn the techniques as well.

COPYRIGHT

Disclaimer:

Shak Stroke therapy is to be considered an addition to the many different methods of helping to heal Stroke survivors / head trauma survivors

Physiotherapy is a major factor in the correction of limb / muscle / tendon movement and works very well with Shak Stroke therapy!

Never stop your prescribed medication once you feel the very fast benefits of Shak Stroke therapy, always consult the person who prescribed the medication and only allow these people to alter the dosage as they **and they only** deem fitting to your condition

Remember: Every single individual is totally unique, as is stroke and Brain related ailments. Although Shak works well on many, it may not work on some, who have very <u>severe</u> Brain damage! Shak has helped to improve some quite sever injuries, purely because the individual was able to barely latch on to the human voice and the instructions given. This may not happen in all cases!

TABLE OF CONTENTS

CHAPTER ONE

The author and founder of Shak Therapy: John Wilson Green: studied hypnosis techniques since 1974: founder of Shak Therapy

My name is *John Wilson Green*, born Thursday April 16th 1959 07.30am; in the upstairs front master bedroom of number 3 Tyne Street, Hessle road Hull, East Yorkshire, In my Nana and Granddads king size bed!

At aged around 18 months I was sat on mum and dads bed playing with the lazy light switch (a lazy light used to hang down from the ceiling so that you could turn it off and on without having to get up from your bed due to that fact in those days, there was no such thing as central heating) My Mum and Dad where talking as I was unwittingly unscrewing the lazy light; exposing live wires and it was not long before BANG and I was thrown to the floor lifeless after being electrocuted (even to this day I have a hole in my hand where the live wire touched my skin) Mum had to run down the street to the telephone box to phone an ambulance, while dad managed to revive me.

Since that eventful day, Things have happened to me and continue to do so; to this day, But! That is a different story.

This particular episode in my life I am referring to is regarding a Phone call I received from my Mum in 1986 asking me to go round to see my father as she is worried about him, she said my Father had collapsed at home and a doctor has been to visit him! Mum said the doctor told my father (Then aged 49) that because he works in a factory near to an open door, He was suffering from frozen shoulder? But; Mum wasn't happy about the diagnosis, so I went straight round to see my Father who was laid in bed with no basic cognitive ability (compared to the fast witted man I know my father to be) and absolutely no control or limb movement down my father's entire left side! Even his left side face had dropped and he was showing signs of expressive aphasia.

I put my two fingers into my Fathers left hand and asked him to squeeze them, He was so disorientated that I saw his right hand squeezing its self into a fist. I asked him to focus on his left hand; But! He could not squeeze my hand at all.

I asked my Mum to call an ambulance as I was not happy about the doctors diagnosis regarding a frozen shoulder and as It turned out I was right; my father had indeed had an cerebrovascular accident (CVA) better known as a stroke to the layman (myself included)

My father was kept in hospital for some weeks and had to undergo physiotherapy, He did not like it because he as he felt it was undignified, which for a shy retiring type of person my father is, I am sure he would rather have had a one on one physio; rather than in a shared room!

After a few physios; where I was present with my father, I asked a Physio practitioner; *"what is the benefit of bending dad's limbs back and forth etc."* … She replied *"Gradually the signal will get back to the brain and he will be able to regain control of his own limb movements"* I said *"wont it be quicker to do that straight from the brain?"* she laughed and said *"No that's impossible"*

Now to me words like that are like a red rag to a bull and even more so; where my father's health is concerned I just had a GUT feeling that with my extensive hypnotic skills, I was sure (Thinking outside of the box as it where!) that there could be a way to speed up dads recovery.

On one of my visits to see my father; the phone rang, It was my aunty, my father answered the phone but! Because his speech was still slurred, I took the call, my aunty was referring to an explosion that happened at the nypro chemical plant near the village of Flixborough, North Lincolnshire, England, on 1 June 1974 and how windows (near to her home) where cracked by the explosion that occurred on the opposite side of the river Humber some miles away. It was that conversation that made me think of a **metaphor** that I would like to try on my Stroke survivor volunteers.

And eureka it worked, my volunteers showed massive improvement within seconds; speech came flooding back along with arm and leg movement and from that day they improved as wasted muscle tissue started to gain strength.

It was from this point that I had to develop the metaphor and combine certain other techniques to make this "THING" even more powerful and so I was allowed to experiment on stroke survivors who quite simply had nothing to lose; I could not make them any worse; because they were at their worst when I first met them, so the least I could do was leave them as I found them without any after effects! And thank them for allowing me the chance to test out my experiments.

Now; 30 years later this "THING" has a name that I call "SHAK Therapy" the word SHAK is Latin meaning **to**

remedy and now it is time to share with others; the techniques used to help not only Stroke survivors but all manner of head trauma conditions, some conditions that even I, after all my years as a practitioner, still come across people who; after just one Shak Therapy; recover from some of the worst head trauma conditions and it just looks for all intents and purposes like a miracle right before your very eyes. It is THE; most rewarding service that I believe you can offer anyone and so that you know … *I have never charged anyone* for this service as I consider each one as an experiment and cannot thank my volunteers enough for letting me test new theories.

I'm at a bit of an impasse with my experiments and have perfected my technique to such a point that I am helping far more than those that I cannot help! I don't want to state a percentage of successful therapies BUT! If I was forced too with my arm held up my back I would say 7 out of ten success rate and that is based on some of them had either very bad hearing due to age OR! They quite simply were not bothered and had given up! To; some with receptive aphasia, meaning they are not able to fully understand my words going in, in the order I say them! And so; cannot get my initial metaphor to work for them!

Some of my volunteers have allowed me to film the before and after SHAK Therapy I have done on them! I would like to share a few stories using only the volunteers Christian names, mostly because I never get to know their surnames as these are people I have never met prior to me visiting their homes. Plus I'm never with them long enough to get to know them.

For some of my volunteer's; even the smallest things that we take for granted can appear to be miraculous to the recipient, such as one person wrote to me thanking me and wanting to hug me; because for the first time in years she had been able to move the mouse around her computer as follows:

March 3rd 2010: "Mr. Green,
I just had to write you this evening with some great news! All I can say is a very heartfelt thank you for this effective tool!
I downloaded your module this morning first thing. I did see some immediate effects even with the guided imagery.
*As I wrote you before, I had a stroke 12 years ago, leaving me with a muscle tone imbalance on my right side. After 18 months of rehab therapy and muscle relaxants, I was only able to open and close my right hand. Because of the tone imbalance, that hand cramps terribly and was virtually useless. I can't play piano yet (LOL), but after just the guided imagery (from the downloaded Shak video), the cramps relaxed and I was able to mouse around my computer screen in relative comfort with my right hand **for the first time in 12 years**. Even better, the hand remained relaxed, warm, and uncramped after that intense activity, and remains so to this very moment!*
I'll grant you that this is nothing compared to what I've seen in your videos, but to be pain free and comfortable for the first time in over a decade is nothing short of amazing to me.
Thank you so very, very much. I would hug you if you were here!
Charlotte

This is just one of many emails I have received from people who have taken the next step and actually used Shak therapy on themselves! And better still; they have even seen and read the negative derogatory things (about my Shak therapy) written by *__internet TROLLS__* and yet! Still went ahead and downloaded the Shak self-help video and for that I thank you from the bottom of my heart for trusting in my methods.

Note:

Shak therapy has been released to the world as an alternative therapy for over a decade and just because you have never heard of it, does not mean it's not there!

There are discoveries every single day such as:

Did you know that 441 new species of plants and vertebrates have been discovered in the amazon rainforests in the last four years alone?

Just because you didn't know they existed; doesn't mean they are not real!

I had the tools and knowledge to develop an alternative stroke recovery therapy that really does work and not only works, but! Works very fast on many people who are very glad that they took the leap from traditional methods to try something new to them but! Not new in terms of the amount of years it has been around.

It's only new to you; because you are learning about it here by reading this book.

All that can be asked; is; of course be sceptical... but! Take the leap and don't talk yourself out of it by thinking its another false hope.

I would never do that to people and give false hopes, which would be a sick joke to play on people.

The recoveries I've witnessed still impress me to this day. Check out a few case studies as follows:

CASE 1—MAXINE

In 2009 Maxine was recommended to me by a taxi driver friend of mine; I was asked if I could help her after she had a stroke in 2007 whilst on her vacation in turkey where she initially had a mini stroke (A transient ischaemic attack (TIA) or "mini stroke") and upon arrival back in England Maxine described to me that she had a full blown stroke (cerebrovascular accident (CVA))

I phoned Maxine up to arrange to meet her one week later at her home and told her that there is *no charge* for this service, But! Asked her if I was allowed to film the before and after with my video camera to show others that there is hope for those who have given up trying anymore. (Even if Maxine had refused filming I still continue with therapy)

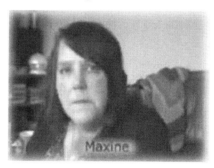

Maxine agreed willingly and explained that she was having fits (seizures) quite frequently, sometimes two or three per day. I spoke to her using some basic metaphors to help calm her down and assured her I will be there to help her recovery speed up dramatically!

When I arrived at Maxine's house as arranged one week later, she looked quite nervous; as many people do when I first visit them, but! This soon passes as we build up a rapport, with humour injected into the conversation. (Humour is very important when performing SHAK therapy).

Maxine's speech was very slow and she was unable to fully pronounce her words without her feeling the need to verbally stretch them and so when she said "Full Blown Stroke" it came out as "ffuuulll bllownnn ssstroke".

The stroke also affected Maxine's right side giving her cause to attend speech therapy classes, the feeling in her right side of the face had all but gone and she could barely lift her right arm or straighten it for that matter

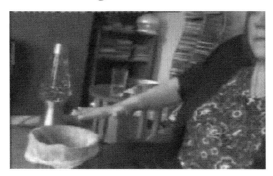

Could not raise arm fully

Maxine could not fully straighten her arm or raise it very high due to the pain it caused.

(Actual video is available to view on YouTube just type in as shown below)

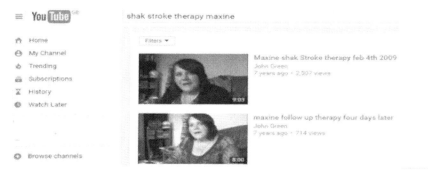

Shak Stroke Therapy Maxine

(Picture below)

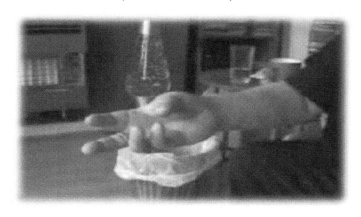

Could not touch thumb to her fingers

When Maxine tried to demonstrate her thumb to finger touching exercise, she had to really focus, she was talking and moving very slowly, again she was in pain doing just that simple movement.

I felt frustration for her and I am sure that many people who are locked in this helpless world of free movement denial; can be... and are; equally as frustrated and understandably depressed at the prospect of a bleak future ahead.

This is why I look forward to doing my Shak therapy on people because it lifts people's emotions through the roof, not only the Stroke survivor themselves but! The onlookers who have on many occasions described what they see as a Miracle.

Maxine said her seizures are happening quite frequently, she said it's funny but; up until last week they were happening once a day, getting the shaking movement's ones and the praying ones? She then said *"Until I talked to you* (over the telephone) *I haven't had one"*

Maxine and I made a note of the time and date which was twenty six minutes past eleven in the morning, February 4th 2009 and **Maxine's first** ever Shak therapy was about to begin, she was quite apprehensive; as most people are when it comes to the unknown but had a glint in her eye and was mentally ready to proceed.

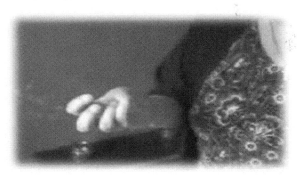

Approximately **15 minutes later** Maxine looked and behaved like a different person!

Her speech was noticeably faster; as was her actions. I asked Maxine *"How does your face feel?"* at which she shot up from her chair, Went over to the mirror hanging on the wall and said *"Have a Look"* She looked at her face in the mirror and said *"Oh WOW!"* as she could visibly see that her right side face had quite literally lifted itself and made her whole face look more balanced.

In the reflection of the mirror you can see her son who is quite taken aback by what he is witnessing his mother doing! I.e. standing up very fast **without** holding on to anything and **quickly** walking across to the mirror to look at her-self!

Maxine lifted her right arm up without any thought of stiffness or pain and then started to touch her thumb to the tip of each finger on her right hand with great ease. Whereas prior to Shak Therapy she could hardly move the right hand and definitely could not touch her finger tips with her thumb! And with that her face lit up smiling happy, she started jumping up and down with sheer excitement and said to her son *"Willy, I can talk"* clapping her hands and repeating *"I can Talk, I can talk"* Her speech since then is improving daily.

Maxine could not stop showing her new found excitement and wanted to give me a hug! She could not stop touching her thumb to each finger; which was even faster!

I asked her son *"Can you see a difference in her"* he replied (with a beaming smile) *"Yeah definitely"*

Depressed

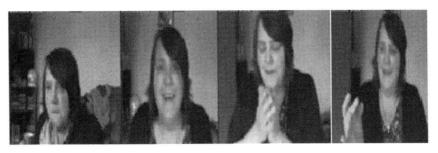

From the first day of meeting to this smiling face in just fifteen minutes

I had my hug off Maxine and left.

This is what makes Shak Therapy very rewarding and contrary to any person who writes derogatory things about me (A person they have never once met) I can assure you that no actors are used and that these lovely people have allowed me to show the world that there is always hope.

A very wise man Called Herbert Spencer wrote: There Is a Principle which is a bar against All Information, which is Proof against all arguments and which cannot fail to keep a man in everlasting Ignorance. That Principle is: <u>Contempt Prior to Investigation</u>

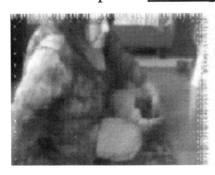

Sits on the floor

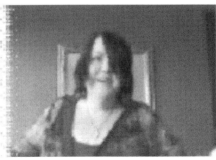

Gets up unaided

Four days later I went back to Maxine's home for a follow up and a catch up and was greeted by a smiling happy lady at the door, who looked nothing like she was when I first visited her! Maxine was cheerful jolly happy excited and could not wait to show me how she can now sit down on the floor and get back up again without having to hold onto things for balance etc.

I was very impressed by the total persona change; from a very depressed looking person to this lovely happy woman wanting to show herself off to the world.

Maxine's speech is improving daily and she can now raise her right arm above her head without hardly any effort.

Now Maxine can sit on the floor from a standing position and get back up again unaided

Maxine has a chart to fill in whenever she has a seizure, she showed it to me and it had <u>one</u> box filled in where she felt a seizure coming on but! She managed to stop it.

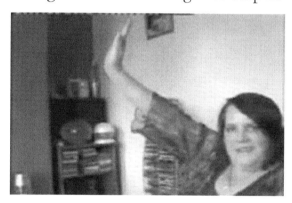

Arm raised above head

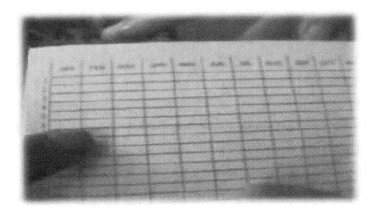

One box ticked

Also during our brief chat Maxine mentioned that she had a dizzy spell and has to write these down in her diary. She showed me the hand writing in her diary for a specific reason… The reason being is that she felt compelled to use her right hand to write it with, the hand that she had lost control over; for two years. Maxine wrote with her right hand. This to me was very exciting; to see the knock on effects that Shak Therapy can produce. It's a blessing in disguise.

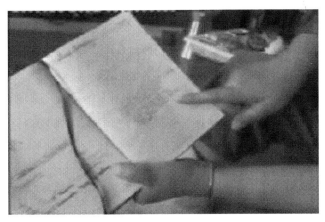

Written with her right hand

There is clearly a magnificent change in Maxine and she constantly kept saying thank you… But! Really I need to thank Maxine and people like Maxine who have allowed me to capture on video; the before Shak therapy and after! For without these lovely people showing others that there is a light at the end of the tunnel; there would be less people wanting to carry on.

CASE 2—MARION

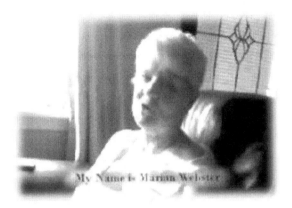

My Name is Marion Webster

In 2012 I had a phone call from a man named Ted; who asked if I would call round to his home to try Shak therapy on his wife Marion who has had pain and restricted mobility for five years since her Stroke! I arranged a day to visit Marion and went to her home.

Ted let me in and introduced me to his wife Marion who was sat in her chair near to the front bay window, looking quite down and fed up with herself! I asked Marion for permission to use the video so that others can see that there is a light at the end of the tunnel. She willingly agreed!

I asked Marion to say to the camera, the reason why I am here. Marion replied *"The reason John is here to help me with pain and hopefully a little bit of better mobility than I've got"*

I moved the camera down to show Marion's left hand witch was in a constant spasm, she said it is quite bad with spasms and if she relaxes it, it just wants to twitch all the time! Like a spider on its back.

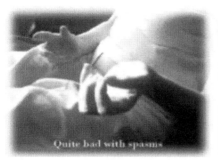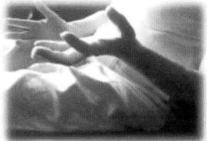

Left hand is constantly twitching.

I pointed the camera to her left foot and saw the toes curled into what can only be described as a claw like position and locked like that for the last five years!

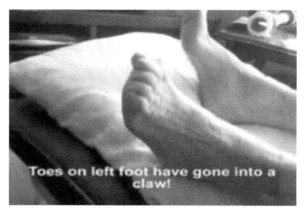

Toes locked in a claw position for five years

Marion said she is quite literally walking on her toe nails sometimes and has to keep them cut short otherwise she is walking on her toenails and is so painful!

I asked Marion *"on a scale of one to ten; how much pain are you in?"* she replied *"I would say seven or eight"*

At this I just wanted to get straight onto actually doing a Shak therapy to alleviate her pain, I don't actually need to know every symptom; because Shak therapy has a very good knock on effect, Kind of like a domino effect; you start at one end and the rest just fall into place; as I was about to find out with Marion!

Ted, (Marion's husband) had gone out to pick up their daughter and so was unaware of anything Marion was having done to her.

I did a Shak Therapy on Marion which (on this occasion), took around twenty five minutes to do.

Just as I had completed Marion's first (and ONLY) ever Shak therapy, Ted came back in and was astonished at how different his wife was looking.

Marion was stood up saying she feels absolutely brilliant and said I want you to look at my toes now!

I lowered the camera to her left foot and saw her toes more relaxed and flat on the floor! Marion was amazed saying *"They were bent right under"* I said *"do they feel any better?"* Marion replied *"Well I've got a box full of shoes I can wear now"*

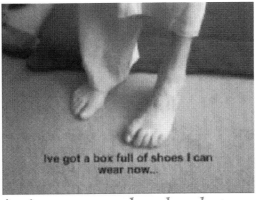

Ive got a box full of shoes I can wear now...

Marion's toes now relaxed and opened up

Marion showed me her left hand which has now stopped having spasms and said she has now got more control over it, Ted said she would grip his hand tight and hurt because it just spasmed and gripped involuntary.

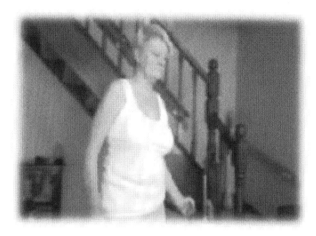

Posture much straighter

Another thing Marion and Ted both noticed was how much straighter her posture is, Ted said *"she is much straighter now!"*

Marion said her sciatic pain has now gone! She said her face is a lot straighter. I mentioned her jaw ache… she said that's gone at which Ted said "No Earache?" Marion toucher her ear and said "No funnily enough, that's gone as well"

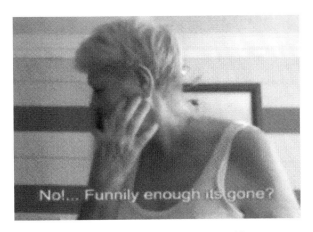

Jaw ache and ear ache totally gone

As the minutes went on Marion and husband Ted where both noticing the things that have suddenly changed since Marion had her Shak Therapy!

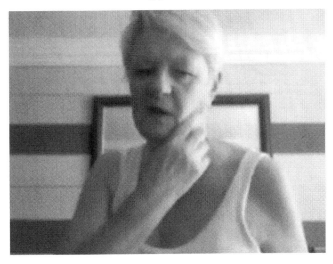

Marion said that the skin on her face even hurt her and that has stopped too!

Skin no longer hurts on Marion's face!

I was thanking Marion for allowing me to film her so that others can see the difference from the before to the after shots when Marion said *"There is a life after a stroke; believe me!"* … Just as I was about to stop filming, Marion lifted her trousers leg up to reveal her left knee saying *"Do you know what! My knee's going straight as well!"*

Ted said he thought she had arthritis in her knee and now realises it isn't, he said *"I think it wasn't arthritis, I think it was the stroke"* Marion demonstrated by bending her left leg slightly saying *"That leg was like that, but! Now is back to normal"*

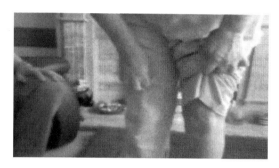

Left leg has straightened up

Marion walked across the room saying "I just can't believe it"… when Ted asked her to hold his hand with her left hand, she held his hand at which Ted said *"Before she would actually have really clenched hard and she didn't know she was doing it"* Marion replied *"It wasn't me though that was doing it Ted it was the spasm that was doing it"*

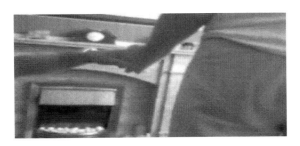

No longer hurting her husband's hand when holding it

Marion sat down and husband Ted went over to her and held her toes on the left foot, He started to rub them saying *"does that hurt you?"* Marion said *"No it doesn't Ted"* followed by *"Before he couldn't touch them"*.. Ted was very surprised and was bending and straightening her toes… Marion said *"They are so supple"* Ted said her left foot used to twist inwards (like a pigeon toed persons) and that has even straightened itself out.

I asked Marion to try to describe the pain she was in prior to me arriving half an hour earlier! She said *"I could imagine it to be like a body full of broken bones!"*

She said the pain in her hip has gone, the pain in her ribs has gone, sciatic pain has gone. Marion started wriggling her toes and Ted said *"she couldn't do that before!"*

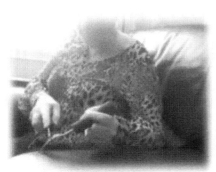 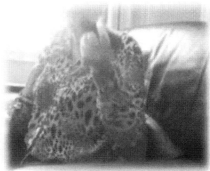

USING A KNIFE AND A FORK

Four days later I went back to see Marion and Ted and Marion was very uplifted and wanted to tell me that she wasn't able to use a knife and fork prior to the Shak Therapy, but! Said; "Tuesday *night; Ted did me a little bit of tea and I used a knife and fork, I couldn't believe I was doing it!*" she added *"Even he couldn't believe it!*" she added *"I was so fussy"*

Marion said that since being able to use a knife and fork again; it makes her feel a bit more human now!

Marion lifted her left foot to show she was wearing actual shoes!

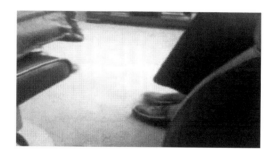

WEARING SHOES AGAIN

Marion said she is not flicking her leg anymore when she walks and that her toes are now bending as she is walking! She is very impressed with how flexible things are becoming now!

Marion said to Ted over the last three days she said *"I don't know what he's done, but! He's done something?"*

I told Marion that I get people on the internet saying it's a con and I'm a phoney etc... Marion replied *"SEND THEM TO ME"*

Ted said *"That's living proof, because I've had to live with it for five years"*

I cannot thank Marion and Ted enough for allowing me to publicise my visit with them and wish them well for the future!

Find the YouTube video; just type in the wording shown below

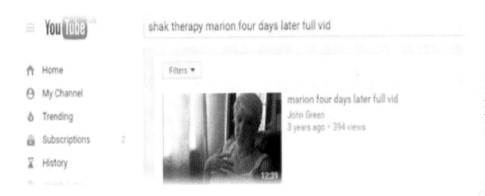

CASE 3—TONY

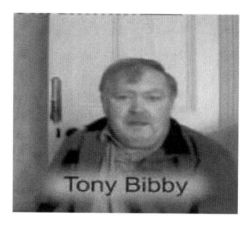

Tony Bibby

In 2009 I went to visit a very lovely man named Tony Bibby who contacted me via some phone numbers I had on an old website.

Tony told me that he had a Stroke august 2006 and was given 3 days to live and was told that when he came out of the coma (after five and a half weeks) that he would very unlikely be able to move his left arm or left leg again! He added that he has proved the doctors wrong and has got SOME movement in his left hand and can manage to touch the first three fingers with his thumb; but cannot touch the little finger at all.

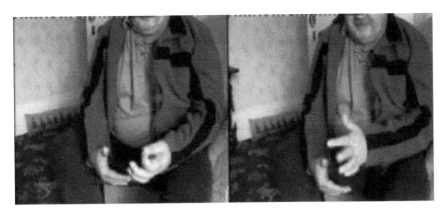

Left hand has some movement but not full control

Tony said that as he focuses his mind on his left hand to touch the fingers, the right hand tries to follow!

I asked tony *"how is your memory?"* Tony replied *"I used to own a company, I no longer own a company; obviously that's gone by the by"* he added *"and I suppose I do feel a bit upset about that!"* he added *"but I'm not capable... I can't read any more..."I used to be a bit of a bookworm, I used to love my archaeology and my history"* I asked Tony to describe why he cannot read anymore? Tony replied *"If I read a first line; I start reading it; but! By the time I get the first line finished, it starts becoming a bit foggy what I've actually been reading"* he added *" so memory wise, I can't recall what I've been reading"* he added *"My daughter gave me a book to read and I'm averaging two lines a day!"*

I thanked Tony for the brief chat and told him I would stop filming and the next time I switch on the camera will be after the Shak Therapy!

Approximately **8 to 10 minutes later** I turned on the camera and viewers can clearly see a different face looking at the camera. Initially the look of confusion; followed by a smile, followed by the urge to do something that He has not been able to do unaided (for three years) nor wanted to do prior to the shak therapy and this is just GET UP AND WALK un aided.

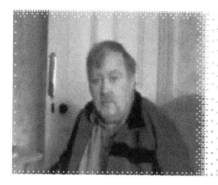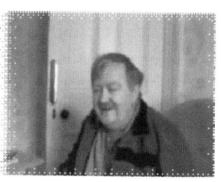

Confusion   *followed by a*   *confident smile*

I said to Tony, "You've had a very brief Shak experience and can you describe how you are feeling since before and after?" Tony replied "I don't really know how to say it, I don't know how to feel it" he added "But! I want to stand up!" he added "erm... I certainly didn't want to stand up before!" and the without any effort at all, Tony stood up and started walking to the middle of the room.

As Tony was walking he said "I can't really believe the way it's making a difference"

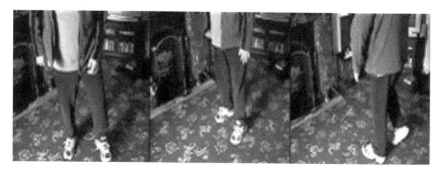

Walking unaided turning around lifting left leg up and down

Tony stopped, turned around unaided and said *"I don't know if I'm actually walking improving or not? But! it makes me feel like I can stand up and move around!"* he started lifting his left up and the right leg then the left leg up and down saying *"I couldn't lift this leg up and do this!"* he added *"I certainly couldn't walk on the spot"*

I asked *"what about your left arm?"* tony lifted the arm and said *"I'm touching my finger tips and I've just managed to touch the fourth one; which I haven't been able to do even before the stroke, So I'm impressed with this!"*

Off camera I asked Tony to read something out of a book for me and since the Shak therapy; I asked Tony about his reading ability now!

Tony replied *"I've just read the first line on a page; and I can actually understand what I've just read and I've never done that for three years"* I asked for permission to show the world and Tony gladly said yes!

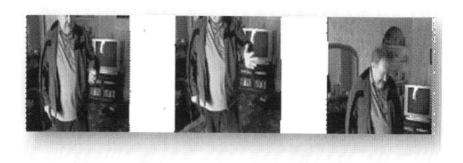

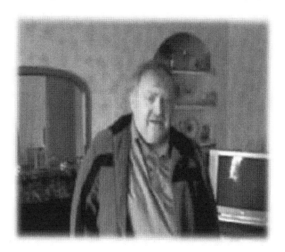

Mr Tony Bibby

It is a real pleasure being able to help; not just the lovely Tony Bibby but! all of the people who have allowed me to continue my experiments, which I hasten to add are not in any way harmful and do help me to improve my techniques as each case is dependently unique, I would like to say one method suits all, but! It doesn't, what I will say; is that anyone can learn what I have developed and I am willing to share this with you.

It is something that will benefit so many people around the world and I have had people fly from all over the world just to meet me and have shak therapy done and gone home smiling again.

My testimonials from my DVD have been glowing, which spurs me on.

I will show one more case before I move onto the methods that I use.

You can find Tony Bibby Video on YouTube by typing in the wording below.

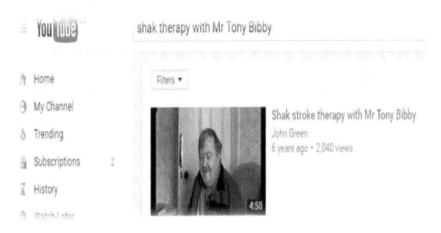

CASE 4--ANGIE

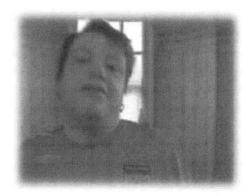

This is Angie, who I have known a number of years and have helped with mobility after her having seven strokes over the years.

Prior to this story I'm about to write! I must tell you a serious and yet! Had a funny outcome; story; about Angie after one of her more serious damaging strokes that she had.

I used to own a bar and bed and breakfast (better known as a B & B in England) when I had a phone call from a person who I; at first could not understand because the speech was so slurred and slow, It took me a short while to realise that is was Angie on the phone and she was saying "Help Me" I said "Have you had another stroke" she replied that she had indeed had, (a month earlier) a massive near death episode. I could barely understand her and as I could not leave my business unattended, I asked if she could get to me somehow? She said yes and a short while later arrived in a taxi.

The driver had to physically lift Angie onto her feet and support her entire weight on his shoulder to keep her from falling, I ran over to assist and sat Angie down in my bar area on a seat near to the door. The Taxi driver left a little exhausted for want of a better word.

I have never seen Angie this bad before and to be very honest, was not sure If my Shak therapy would work on her this time because she could not even lift her own head up, nor move any part of her left side, she was actually falling to her left side and could not put her arm out to stop herself from hitting the floor! I had to totally support her from falling forwards or sideways.

A member of my staff called Andy was cleaning my bar and I asked him to go for a tea break so that I could have some privacy with Angie!

I said to Angie... *"I'll make you a deal, I will do this on one condition and no ifs or but's..."* I added *"I'll only do this if you agree to never have any more cigarettes ever again, because it's going to kill you and I don't want that."* Angie nodded her head in agreement.

Now as I said, I have never seen Angie this bad (not fully sure if she was compos mentis I suppose?)

I just hoped that she was able to fully understand me and was not suffering from any receptive aphasia.

I nervously continued with a shak therapy. I was totally blown away at how rapidly she came back to reality, latching onto her limbs and reflex movements all within minutes and quite literally lifted her head and said *"Oh that's better, it's my cousin Julies birthday and I wanted to be there, she thinks I can't go because of my stroke, but! Now thanks again to you*

I'll be able to go and surprise her!" I called my staff member Andy back in and asked if he could call the same taxi service that Angie used to bring her and asked specifically if the very same driver could come for her! Andy was puzzled watching Angie walking up and down flicking her legs saying wow and other excited words that I cannot write her.

A short time later the Taxi cab pulled up outside my Bar and even parked onto the kerb as near to my door as he could; so that Angie didn't have too far to be <u>carried</u> (I suppose) I jokingly said to Angie, you sit there and I'll ask the driver to come in for you, which she did.

I went outside and (with a serious face) said *"she's ready if you want to come and get her"* The driver came in and Angie just stood up smiling said *"thank you"* to me and shook the driver's hand and walked un aided to the waiting taxi cab.

The look of total confusion on the drivers face was priceless, he started looking up and around and actually said *"what is this, like a candid camera show"* to which Andy my staff member replied *"that's what I thought too!"* Angie and the driver left and a few days later Angie's cousin Julie came in (very emotional) Gave me the biggest hug saying *"I don't know what you did?, But! I cannot thank you enough, seeing Angie walking through the door on my birthday was my birthday gift from you"* at which Andy my staff member interrupted saying *"Don't you think John's weird"* ha ha Julie hugged me and said *"You leave him alone"* all in good humour of course.

I digress… On this particular occasion 22nd January 2009; I went to visit Angie at her Public house, she had; had a stroke which left her left side uncontrollable as well as affected her speech.

I asked Angie to walk towards me and could clearly see that she was dragging and flicking her left leg which clearly made her balance very shaky indeed. I asked her *"How's your balance"* she replied *"Not good"* I then said *"If I said to you say A B C D E F G... can you do it?"* Angie's head went up and backwards and she had difficulty not only remembering the alphabet, But! Was slurring each letter as well as constantly wiping her mouth?

I said I was making a note of the time which was exactly four pm.

I asked Angie to lift her least useful; at which; she pointed to the left arm and wriggled her fingers. She lifted her good arm first and wriggled her fingers, I said now; do it with the other arm! Angie made a very strenuous effort to raise her arm and could barely lift it; her left hand was like a claw; fingers together like a scoop on a JCB digger, limp wristed and for all intents and purposes, pretty useless!

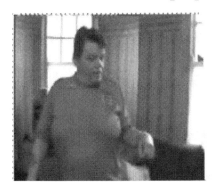 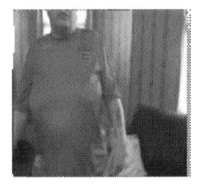

(Having difficulty raising her left arm)

Angie said *"it won't go up"* I said "Is it not lifting up at all?" Angie gave her best effort once again to lift her left arm, but! Again it was very difficult for her to do! She said in a slurred voice whilst wiping her mouth continuously *"It's heavy"* I said to Angie *"also you keep wiping your mouth, why do you do that?"* she replied *"because I feel as though I'm slavering"*

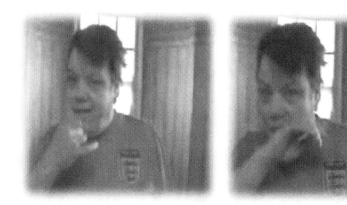

(Constantly wiping her mouth)

I asked Angie *"How does your face feel?"* She rubbed her right side of her face and said it's fine this side" I said "what about the other side?" Angie rubbed her right hand to left side of her face, started pulling at the skin and said "Just…Fat" which made us both laugh at the description she gave.

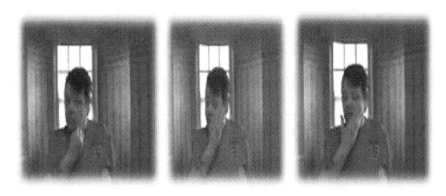

(Pulling on her face, said it feels like fat)

At that point I switched off the camera to do a Shak therapy on Angie and approximately eight minutes later she was all done and finished.

I switched my camera back on and in plain view; you can see Angie sat on the sofa smiling and rubbing her legs with BOTH hands.

I asked Angie if she wouldn't mind standing up for me, which she did willingly in one smooth motion; straight up and onto her feet without any wobbling or correction needed.

I asked her to walk towards me, Stop turn around and walk the other way, which she did. I said *"and stop, Turn the other way"* Angie did this perfectly with great control, compared to a few minutes earlier.

I asked Angie to lift the arm that she couldn't lift earlier and touch her face with it; Angie lifted her left arm with ease and rubbed the left side of her face! I asked *"and how does your face feel now?"* Angie replied *"Face feels great now"* I said *"Feel good?"* Angie replied *"Yes"*

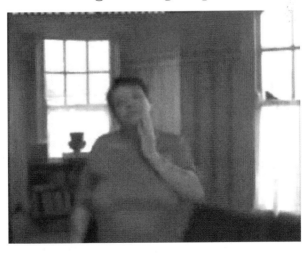

I asked Angie if she would now say the alphabet, which she did in a clear fluent voice without any signs of struggling to get the words out!

Angie was stood there smiling and we noticed that her face was all balanced out as it should be.

Angie started flicking her feet rubbing her arms and face and said *"I'm here!"*

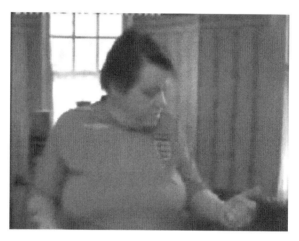

(Confused but Happy!)

Just before I turned off the camera, Angie lifted her left arm, rubbed it and said *"Wow"*

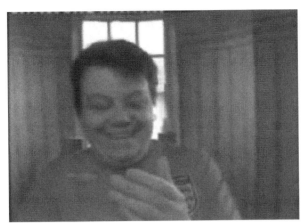

(Look of happy astonishment at getting movement back in her left arm)

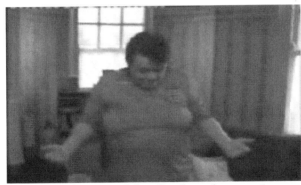

(Amazed at how quickly she has been given control over her body again!)

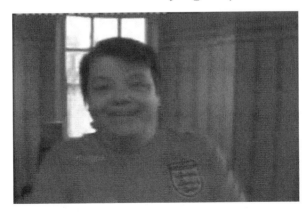

(Happy again)

(You can find Angie's YouTube video by typing in the wording below)

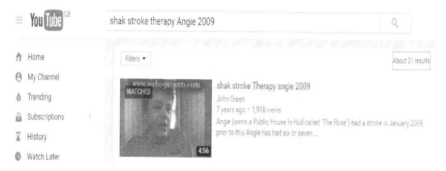

Over the 30 years of developing Shak therapy I have met and helped hundreds of people; who have very kindly allowed me to experiment on them and I cannot thank these lovely people enough.

As I have stressed whilst writing this, I have never charged a single person for Shak therapy

I have left the bar business and make my living as an entertainer to pay my bills and keep a roof over my head!

My goal is to open up a walk in clinic and get away from the entertainment industry, of which I've been a part of for over forty years! I am hoping that this book will generate enough funds to achieve my goal of running seminars for groups who want to learn; hands on; How to become a Shak practitioner, So that there can a trained person in every single part of the world, able to help not only Stroke survivors, but! Head and trauma survivors too! Etc.

I have used the same methods that can give limited but! Valued and very welcome pain relief for arthritic pain and **Osteoarthritis** pain, with amazing results, this method I named Aargon which means pain gone in Latin.

I had to give these methods names; otherwise they would mean and be nothing to anyone but! A; *"John Green can help you!"*

In my younger days I was a stage hypnotist and found that I prefer clinical therapy more than making people into chickens laying egg in front of audiences. I prefer the healing therapeutic side; which gives me far more pleasure seeing happy smiling faces.

Throughout my life I believe that the words caring and sharing are what we humans are here for, to care enough to share what we learn and pass it on to the next generation who undoubtedly will improve on it and possibly even make a hologram to simplify the teaching methods. (Who knows what will become of our ideas now?)

I have taken a very long break from doing any form of shak therapy due to the bombardment of negative internet trolls calling me a fraud and saying I am ripping my volunteers off with money? (Although I've never charged one person I personally have done a shak therapy too!) It was affecting my private life and my partner said I needed to pull away from these people, so I did; just for sanity reasons. How these people are allowed to get away with these derogatory remarks about someone they have never met, nor ever contacted as they claim? It sickens me at the thought of how many people could have had far better lives after their Strokes and head trauma, if these internet trolls had just left me alone to get on with my work.

Recently I decided to write about my experiments and how to teach others the methods I use; that have worked for me and hopefully someone will take my methods and improve on them to fine tune them even more than I have done thus far!

I'm now going to teach you how to become a shak therapist!

I made a video in 2007 explaining about Shak Therapy and showing exactly how I perform it on others.

I will transcribe the entire video whilst adding anything I feel needs to be added for you the reader.

The video opens with me explaining about shak therapy.

CHAPTER 2

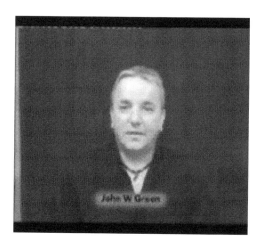

Opening shot

John Green: "Hello and welcome to the world of shak therapy, my name is John Green" … "Shak therapy; must not ever be confused with the miracle cure, It isn't a miracle cure, it's a means to help the mind understand how to divert signals around a damaged area! Dependent upon how damaged the area is; will depend upon how the person can actually understand you! So; it depends on the receptiveness. If they are very receptive and; understand everything clearly; it makes this particular therapy a lot easier.

So! Shak therapy, what does it do... it stimulates areas of the brain; areas of the mind that the once depressed person; thought that they were trapped inside of! It helps to open up and unlock new avenues, new ways of getting these signals around the brain; to start to make the persons limbs; function again! Dependent upon how good their imagination is; depends upon how well the shak therapy will work.

So what we need to do is to actually stimulate their imagination; by using metaphors and these metaphors are very powerful! The metaphor that we use for shak therapy; has been so powerful; it doesn't need to have any other metaphor! So please; when you watch the video / the DVD; listen to the metaphor.

Write your own metaphor based around the areas you live; so the person your going to give the shak therapy too; will actually understand and relate to what you are talking about.

A metaphor; is a story about something that seems to be totally far away from the subject matter; but! As you start listen to the story; it actually relates to what we are talking about; in a different way, But! It stimulates the mind in such a way; that it will start to form pictures and it will start to understand better without being direct and without being rude! It's a very very crafty way; a sly way; of getting the message across to the deep side of the unconscious mind! Where the unconscious mind will suddenly go! "I know what you're talking about, I understand now… YES! Why didn't anybody tell me this before?" (A light bulb moment as it where)

And now; we are going to instil something else, which is excitedness, you must be excited when you are doing shak! You MUST be excited; you must be passionate about it; you must, you be; almost as if you are climbing inside that persons brain and giving all them all the stimulation and the excitement that your feeling and the more that you do this particular shak therapy on people; the more you will understand how clever it does work; it's pretty crafty (means sneaky) it's pretty crafty.

Some people are so depressed that they don't want to talk to you! They just do not want to know you; whatsoever! (You must think to yourself) SO WHAT! Just get in there! Just talk, Use the metaphor; they will look at you with confusion, they'll look at you as if you're an alien; But! Keep talking... It doesn't matter! GET THROUGH THAT BARRIER.

The next part of shak is touch!

Touch, It's quite amazing but! If a stranger; touches you on your shoulder, the first thing that will happen is; your unconscious mind will direct you straight to this area and effectively you're in a state of trance! Your unconscious mind is at the forefront, your conscious mind; has just lost its analyticalness for a moment, your unconscious mind has gone *"ooh... Feel?"* because the sense of feel will go direct to your unconscious mind.

But! If you've had a stroke or some form of traumatic damage to a particular area, you may not be receiving those signals, now! Prior to touch; you have just given a metaphor, this metaphor has suddenly; changed the way the mind thinks! Your excitedness is also changing the way the person is feeling, the person now; is feeling pretty excited although confused... still pretty excited and now you're about to instil touch on top of all this! This is mind blowing, quite literally; it's going to stimulate areas of the mind; that at one time you though you could not stimulate, you thought you could not get in there... You've got in there already! The metaphor has diverted signals around the damaged area, Treating it almost as a roundabout; like car's go around a roundabout! Well this is what's happening now! These signals are being diverted everywhere and suddenly the persons feeling's that they couldn't feel in; thumbs, In tongue (speech impaired) and the side of the face, Start to become; re-energised, re-vitalised, Just by talking, Now! Added with the sense of touch; this is so mind blowing, the unconscious mind is saying "I want more, I want more; tell me more; show me more!"... You're getting excited, you're doing this (what you are about to be show) you're copying exactly what is going to be shown to you! The excitedness from your voice, Is almost as if you are that other persons subconscious mind! You're excitedness will become; THEM! It will instil into that person; so much, they're just overtaken and now; this is a form of hypnosis! Even though we are not talking about hypnosis! It is a form of hypnosis; whether you like it or not? You're attaching yourself; you mirror and match Mirror and match! Then you start to lead and pace and now you are leading and pacing, you are the joystick for this person in front of you! And they are getting pretty excited, because they're actually genuinely feeling; these tingly feelings; in areas that they couldn't feel before (before they met you) and the nice thing is, If the side of the face has been dropped for years, Right before your eyes and in front of the people that are watching (amazed) baffled confused but! Amazed! You will see the face start to lift up! Start to balance... It's fantastic; it's such a lovely thing to watch, it has been described as a miracle! Now! It's going to happen in some cases; phenomenally fast and very very big and prominent. It's going to happen in other cases, very slow; But! It will start to show a difference, It will start to show a change in the person! Once you have started to show a change, give it a week, Let their mind settle again, let them get all settled again, then do it again a week later! You'll notice that there's more change, but! the good thing is; the person is actually excited about you coming to see them! They've got something to look forward too at last! So use shak to help people! Help as many people as you can! Spread the word around, use shak! It is very very powerful! The metaphor that we use; relating to the (geographical) area we live in, works fantastic for people in the Hull and East Yorkshire area! It works fine, because they can relate to their own area! The metaphor can be changed slightly to suit your own location; it will help people in your own geographical location, because their unconscious mind will relate to that! It also gets the unconscious mind thinking! And drawing pictures! So tell them to use their brilliant imagination, get their imagination so fired up, that by the time they are finished, they are as excited as you and vice-versa! Watch the change in the person! It does work! It's very powerful! Use it wisely! Help people! Share and Care! So please enjoy the rest of the DVD (available online, please send your email address to recoveryfromstroke@gmail.com enjoy the therapy that you're going to be shown, write down notes if possible? And also with the video we'll give you a run-down of the stages that you need to actually go through; when doing a shak therapy, So learn it memorise it, share and care. Thank you.

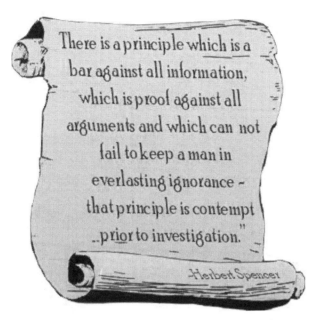

> "There is a principle which is a bar against all information, which is proof against all arguments and which can not fail to keep a man in everlasting ignorance - that principle is contempt ...prior to investigation."
>
> -Herbert Spencer

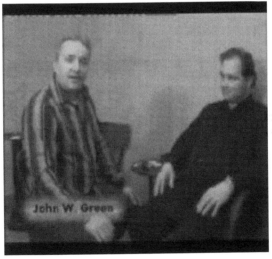

John W. Green

I am going to write word for word, exactly how I am describing how to perform a shak therapy; on my video, which is available as a download.

Visit the website at www.recoveryfromstroke.co.uk

Hello and welcome to shak therapy, My name is John Green and over the years shak has been developed just by trial and error; basically and I've fine-tuned shak into something that everybody can do; whether you know hypnosis or whether you don't know hypnosis; it's irrelevant.

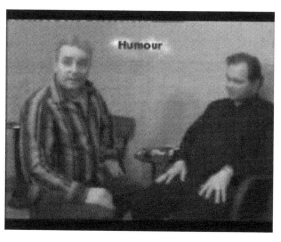

You don't have to understand how the mind works; It does help, but! You don't <u>have</u> to understand how the mind works. All you need to do is follow these simple instructions! Everything is done very very simple; it's done in layman's terms, we like to say it's done A.B.C. 1.2.3! If we teach A.B.C.D. 1.2.3.4! Then we say it's too complicated... So, A.B.C. 1.2.3; is as simple as we need to be with shak.

Now; many people know someone or know of someone; who has had some form of stroke or has some form of disability through an accident; possibly? Maybe they have fallen off a motorbike or something? Shak treatment can improve people a lot! It can bring back sensations that these people at one time; thought they could not get back again. It doesn't work with every person; it all depends on how the nerves have been severed or not severed, it depends on a lot of factors! But! With stroke victims (survivors) most times you won't get 100%, but you will get a vast improvement which is what we are looking for! And that improvement can be improved again and again and again, so you keep improving; on your improvements! So use shak and you'll you can help a lot of people and they can go away and help other people as well!

So what we are going to do (On the video I introduce Jonathan (shown in fig 1) who is purely there to help with a shak demonstration and has not had a stroke or head trauma accident.)

Now shak works primarily on metaphors and you need to be able to speak quite lively quite energetically and very confidently! You can inject <u>humour</u> into the conversation, which does help to alleviate any stresses any awkwardness between yourself and the person who is having the shak treatment.

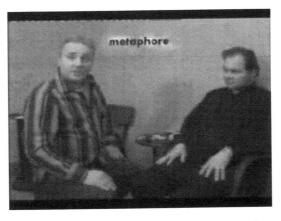

So! What we are going to do is teach you how to use a metaphor, the metaphor we use for the shak treatment; involves a telecommunications system and as this is going out to different countries in the world! What you need to do is work out a script (Supplied at the end of this book for you to fill in the blank spaces!) for yourself to learn based upon; your own country! So you'll understand what I'm saying in a minute; when I mention that here in England; we are based in Hull; as an example and if I go on a telephone in Hull and I phone someone in Leeds: I may go via a telephone exchange in Pontefract! So; as I am talking to the person in Leeds; the signal is going via a telephone communication system in Pontefract; direct to Leeds, It's all done in a millisecond; So! The conversation between me and the person in Leeds is going via another town, Pontefract.

Then all of a sudden, Pontefract telephone exchange; blows up! It just explodes! And in a millisecond, you are instantly diverted to Braford telephone exchange! So you are talking to the person in Leeds; Pontefract blows up; Bradford takes over and in a millisecond; you have no idea that Pontefract has blown up and all you know is that! Your conversation; is still being maintained without any interruptions what so ever; via Bradford! Now your mind starts to understand... "_Send the signal another way_" The metaphor is very powerful, Once the mind starts to understand that is can send a signal via where this explosion is inside the brain; The blockage (The mental blockage) It can send the signal anywhere around (the damaged part of the brain) and it will automatically start to do that once you've instilled this metaphor! So if you live in America for instance you may say; I'm speaking from Florida to Washington via Alabama and Alabama telephone exchange explodes etc. and you get the picture! So use the metaphor that suits your own country! And instil that metaphor into the person; But! Do it quite fast and energetic and lively! The person will look at you almost; with a look of *"what on earth are you talking about"* … That doesn't matter, Just keep doing it, It may feel awkward at first, But! You know the end results are going to help this person! So, just keep doing it and doing it! You're actually talking to the subconscious or the unconscious mind! The conscious mind of that person hasn't got a clue what you are talking about? They don't know why you're even speaking about telephone exchanges! But! The unconscious mind is absorbing this; because it's intrigued, especially if you speak fast! So; speak fast lively energetic and if you can get a cup of tea out of it, that's even better! So… get your nice cup of tea (sip your tea) and talk to this person about a telephone exchange! And once you have got this metaphor through, you'll notice in the person (sat in front of you) a change straight away! Their eyes start to move a lot more! Start to focus; on you! But… as they are focussing on you; their eyes look like they are going dilated, The pupils get wider and their head tilts forward slightly and they sort of look at you upward! Because now; they are starting to feel things happening to their limbs that wasn't getting any feeling before.

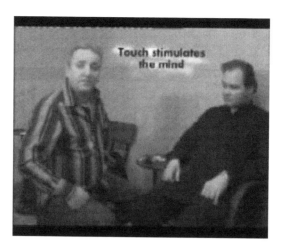

Then we go to part 2, now the unconscious brain is working out this fantastic new thing you've just told them that it can be re-directed; they can send signals all around this damaged area, now it understands; it can be re-directed! So... what we are going to do is send all these signals around the body.

The way we do that is by touch! Once you instil touch; the unconscious mind is more intrigued *"why is this person touching me? I want to know why?"* and what you do is say to the person sat in front of you as I say to Jonathan (my volunteer) now as an example! (Just for the purpose of this exercise) his right arm isn't able to function properly; the right side of his face isn't able to function properly!

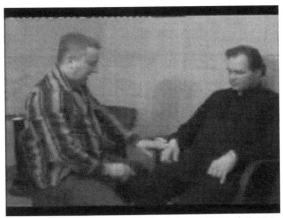

ON A SCALE OF ONE TO TEN

So what I'll say to Jonathan is; "On a scale of one to ten; If I touch you here on your hand (as I tap his hand gently a few times) give me a feeling a rate of how much you can feel me tapping out of one to ten!" Primarily they normally say one or two! I tap the bad hand and say "we need to make that hand (tapping the bad hand) the same as this one" (moving my hand straight across to the good hand) Now on a scale of one to ten (tapping the good hand) ask the person again "On a scale of one to ten, How can you feel me tapping you on this hand?" they'll always say "Ten" which is fantastic! Then we start to do the Magic! The magic is really really good, we say to the person, "what we are going to do is give (tapping the bad hand!) This hand here; the feeling of a ten like this hand (tapping the good hand) this hand (tapping the bad hand) needs to have the feeling of this hand (tapping the good hand) a ten! So we are going to start to do some magic **(the subconscious is intrigued by exciting stimulating words such as; magic and fantastic etc., it comes to the forefront and basically pushes the conscious (analytical) mind to one side and helps to speed up the therapy)**

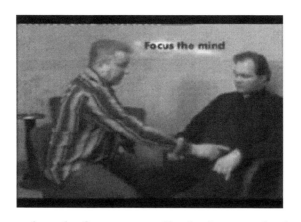

Now remember before; we talked about telephones and how the signals can be diverted; (say to the client) *"I'd like you to focus your mind onto* (tap the hand in time with you speaking) *this hand here and picture that nice feeling of ten"* (as you are talking you are tapping the good hand in a small circular motion as shown in the video) *"The feeling of ten; how you can feel how clear this is!"* Now what you do; is tap and tell the mind to follow your finger, Tell the MIND to follow your finger (say to the client, follow my finger and move it in a tapping motion up the arm in time with your talking... the client will watch you tapping ... then you say to the client *"Follow my finger with your mind, Not your eyes"* this is when they feel a significant change from within themselves) you say "Focus your mind on my finger; I'd like you to follow these feelings and bring these TEN feelings with you all the way around (as your tapping up the arm, Up the side of the face across the top of the head and down the other side) and right through and over; bringing these nice TEN feeling and sometimes when you get about half way down the bad arm, The limb the was quite faulty; May start to jerk in spasms, Don't worry about it; it's just NOW re-energising, Re-vitalising; it will spasm sometimes.

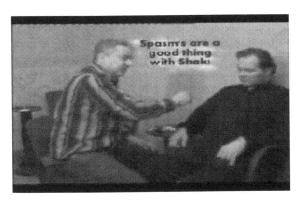

And tap and tap and bring those nice feelings of TEN;
right down to this hand (tapping down the arm and
continue tapping the affected hand... " And the ten
feelings are here (tapping the bad hand) then move across
to the good hand and tap the good hand tap the bad hand
tap the good hand then the bad hand a few times! (With
experience, after doing a few Shak therapies, you can
picture inside yourself the balance that you know you need
for each client; you'll know when it looks and feels right)

TIP: Keep it lively and energetic

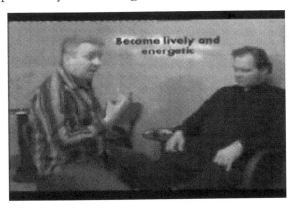

Then say to the client *"On a scale of one to ten, How can you feel
this now?"* (Tapping the bad hand) you will always get a
higher number! ... So it could be six or seven! So we still
need to get TEN. We do it one more time; (Tapping the

good hand, whilst being lively and energetic) saying *"lovely let's get these feelings from here* (tapping the good hand) *and bring the around as your taking these TEN feelings and your mind going to follow me and that fantastic mind is follow me Feeling all of these lovely feelings; taking in a nice deep breath, Feeling re-energised re-vitalised (still tapping as you are speaking) and it's following me, Following me (still tapping) following me right down and into this hand (tapping the defective hand)*

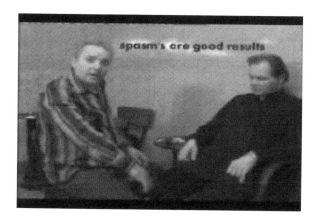

"starting to feel yourself balancing out, feeling yourself balancing out" Sometimes as I said; the hand will spasm as shown in the video, Just let the spasm continue for a while and then say "In a minute; I'm going to touch you and you'll feel it balancing out; just touch the hand tapping slower and slower as the spasms get slower and slower and the client will start to become quite normal and in control!

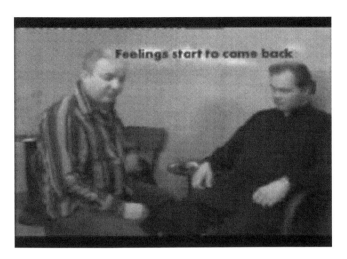

Whilst all of the above is happening, you may notice that the client's facial muscles have lifted up on people who have had a stroke, so the facial muscles start to rise up; without you even doing anything! They will start to chew on their tongue (as feelings flood back into it again) if they have had a speech impediment that has been caused by the stroke, they may start chewing their tongue (video demonstrates how) which is quite normal, it's just that they are getting their sensations back, they are starting to feel the feelings; back in their tongue again and starting to be in control of their own tongue.

The facial muscles have lifted up; their eyes start to sparkle, They are now looking at you as if you are some sort of a weirdo, Which is Great; it doesn't matter, Let them do that!

Then we tap the once bad hand and say *"On a scale of one to ten; how can you feel that?"* (Normally after three goes at this) You normally get a ten! You'll get a balance of both sides (of the body and mind) then we ask the client to rub their own face with the once bad arm onto the once bad side of the face! They will rub their own face and actually be able to feel their face clearly. (This can be quite an emotional experience for some who have been immobile for some years) They can feel their own arm, At last it belongs to them again, it's part of them, it is them it's their arm! The excitement now is getting to both parties (You and the client are getting more excited at the changes occurring) so again tapping the once bad hand, we say *"On a scale of one to ten how do you feel"* and the client will invariably say a higher number; Nine or Ten, I will keep doing the process until I get them onto a TEN! So now I've got a ten and the client is feeling balanced out.

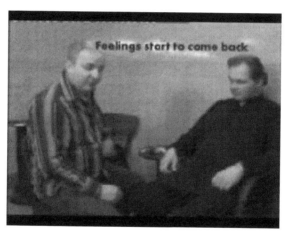

Even though my volunteer on the video has nothing wrong with him, the demonstration shown has actually given him a feeling of clear headedness! Which it does for my clients too; who are genuine stroke and head trauma survivors!

Shak therapy does work, it relieves stress, it relieves every day stresses and strains of the day. Get someone to do it to you and balance yourself out; relieve the stress, take away the strain!

Now that we have sorted out the clients TOP PART of their body, we need now to focus on the legs.

But! This is where the magic starts! Because instead of tapping all around the body, we can do a shortcut and you say to them (now that their subconscious mind is now intrigued in you and your voice and the excitement you are giving them, they know you are fully competent and you are going to help them; with the problem they had prior to you arriving at their house.

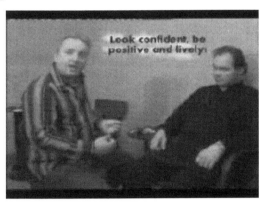

So we tap the bad leg and say *"on a scale of one to ten; how can you feel this leg?"* they will normally say two or a three! Then say "well we want to make this leg feel as good as this leg (tapping the good leg) *"on a scale of one to ten, how can you feel this leg?"* and they will always say TEN because it's the good leg! Then say "good! Because we are going to do a little bit of magic now and this is where the magic starts (tapping the good leg) say *"I'm going to touch this leg and you can start to focus that wonderful mind* (tapping the good leg) *onto this feeling here that I'm giving you, A feeling of TEN; TEN; TEN; but this time we are going to go to this hand here"* (start tapping the good hand) and we are going to JUMP across and your EYES are going to follow me! *"Follow me with your eyes... ready"* (move your hand across to the bad hand which is now a good hand!) saying *"follow across here"* (start tapping the bad side) saying "lovely, bringing that nice feeling of TEN down to here (tap very quickly down to the knee of the bad leg) a lot of times there will be a lot of spasms / spasaming; this is as the nerve endings are coming back to life and there's energy going into that leg and it's also attaching itself to the unconscious mind; becoming part of you again; part of who you are! So once we have repeated the good leg to bad leg (jumping across) a couple of times, the excitement your giving in your voice is instilling into the unconscious mind, it feels fantastic it feels great!

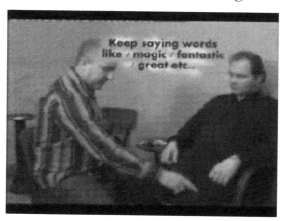

You must talk fantastic great feelings UP; UP; UP; UP; everything's UP; UP! You must be positive in everything that you do! Even in everyday life, be positive; be positive in everything that you say to other people; instil that positiveness in them by talking fast and energetic and being lively, This is what it requires; positiveness! Once you have balanced the person out; just say to them "On a scale of one to ten; how can you feel this leg? ... They say ten... Then tap the once bad hand and again say "On a scale of one to ten; how can; you feel this, they normally say ten!" ... Then you say to them "just take a nice deep breath and I'd like you to stand up and walk across the room!

They'll get up and they won't limp (Most of the time) if they are still limping a little bit; that's only because of wasted muscle tissue; depending upon how long they have had this particular condition, But! They will improve.

MEDICATION ADVICE

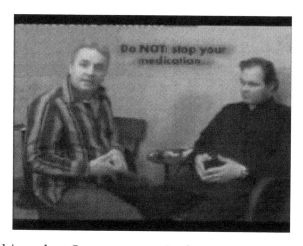

Now a thing that I must stress! If you are on medication; <u>do not</u>! <u>**(Under any circumstances) stop taking that medication; do not stop taking the medication;**</u> you must see your doctor; who will take you off the medication at <u>**the required rate!**</u> They'll be quite impressed on your improvement; but! Once you've been on medication; there is a weening off period that you need to go through your doctor with and they are the only ones that can ween you off this particular medication! So please; don't think "Oh I feel fine now; I'm going to stop taking the medication! You still need to take the medication that is prescribed, to keep the blood thinner; to stop any more clots that may want to form, so please; do everything that your GP (general practitioner) says.

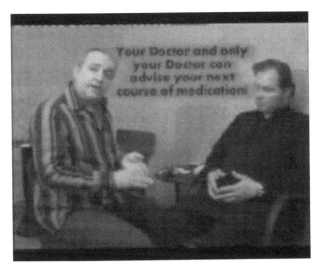

This (meaning Shak Therapy) will make you feel fantastic; it will make you feel a lot better; in most cases! And in a lot of cases, you will see a <u>vast</u> improvement! So; do it; (meaning a shak therapy) give it a week, Do it again! Give it a week; you will see a lot of improvement.

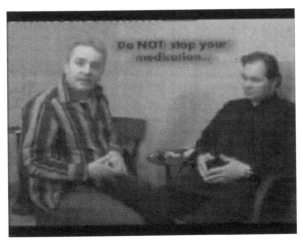

Now! Regarding the wasted muscle tissue! Keep doing the physio's exercises; that's all you need to do.

So! As fast as I have been talking; (writing) is as fast as you have just learnt how to do a Shak therapy! It will improve a lot of people's lives, so please go on and show other people how to do it! Pass it around the world.

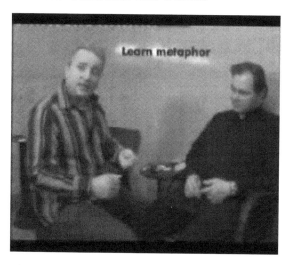

More people need to know how they can help other people! Use it in your repertoire if you are a hypnotherapist, use your own experiences of having had it done (to yourself) learn a metaphor that suits your country; with the telephones and go ahead and help other people. Make people happy

SHARE AND CARE

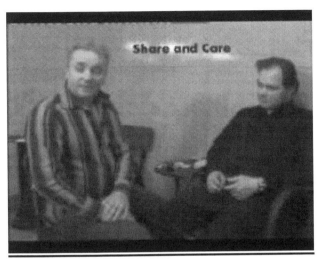

Share and Care

Now it's Your turn to perform a shak therapy

I'm going to break it down as simply as I can

First of all; you will need to learn the initial metaphor in such a way that it corresponds to a geographical area that both you and the Client know! i.e. the first City that is mentioned; is the city that the client lives in, So that they can visualise it comfortably, then pick two nearby cities that the client also knows of!

After a brief chatty rapport, you can suddenly input the metaphor by saying it in a totally **out of context**!) Way; (*away from any subject that you were just talking about*) which causes some mild confusion and helps to bring their now very curious subconscious to the foreground; with a curious need to listen intently at what you are saying! Start off with "*OK let's get the **magic** working; by using this **powerful imagination** Of yours*" (Rub your hands together as if something magic is going to appear before their very eyes) ... saying words like Magic and powerful, will really stimulate the curious side of their imagination; It will bring their whole focus of attention to the forefront and will... on more occasions than not! Effectively open up their subconscious to a very mild trance state, a state that allows input; without the Conscious part of the brain analysing everything and putting any doubt there! The conscious (analytical) part of the brain will effectively nod off out of confusion or boredom and allow the subconscious to take in every suggestion that is given to it... so now *(metaphorically)* the subconscious is the computer that needs a defrag and you are the mouse; moving around clicking at the right time and in the right order.

It is very much akin to a stage hypnotist making their volunteers become chickens laying eggs; or doing other silly things without them even knowing what is happening to them, because they are operating by means of the subconscious part of their brain and the conscious (analytical) part of their brain has been put to sleep; thus allowing you to continue with inputting the necessary guiding instructions that will re-attach motor actions back to the brain!

If you attach a slow droll voice to the subconscious, it will react accordingly and become droll too and get bored; eventually the conscious analytical part of your brain will wake up and not allow you back in, Thus leaving your client exactly how they was before you met them and all trust in your abilities will be gone for good.

You have to approach each person you meet (for Shak therapy) in a very confident; fast paced and slightly humorous way, In order to gain the subconscious mind's attention! To stimulate it into being pleasantly curious about this **stranger** (YOU) who is going to help restore or find new neuro pathways around the brain. The mind learns and is more stimulated when it is taught at a slightly faster pace than normal talk!

Mundane; boring talk loses a person's interest, faster lively energetic talk, engrosses the subconscious mind.

Next I will include the metaphor script both filled in followed by one with blanks for you to fill in using your own geographical locations as follows:

"Shak therapy" Break Down.

The Importance of touch plays a vital part when using Shak Therapy, Touch combined with the right words makes Shak Therapy very powerful indeed!

Make the person receiving Shak therapy feel comfortable and in a warm environment.

Chat to the person in a lively fast jolly (fun) manner to get their unconscious minds attention.

(The conscious part of their brain will wonder who on earth this weirdo is? but! That is quite a normal reaction when performing a **Shak therapy**)

Explain that at some point you will touch the person at this point show them the tip of the finger you will use to touch them with! This puts a trust between you and the person receiving **Shak therapy**

Once a rapport has been attained!

- Input the telephone exchange metaphor!
- Make sure the metaphor relates to locations known to the person receiving **Shak therapy**!
- Use a scale of _**one to ten**_ when tapping the damaged limb area!
- Tell _**the mind**_ to follow your finger all around the good area leading into the damaged areas!
- Sometimes spasms will occur during the **Shak therapy**. This is quite normal and not to be concerned about.
- If spasms occur simply say to the client; when I touch your hand the spasm will come to a stop, gently tap telling the person it is stopping NOW and it will slowly come to a stop.

SIGNS OF IMPROVEMENT

- Keep repeating the Shak therapy until the scale of *one to ten* gets higher!
- Watch for signs of improvement i.e.: the persons face lifts as their muscles start to reactivate.
- The person's speech starts to improve as their tongue begins to regain feeling
- The person's eyes start to look lively and begin to sparkle!
- They start to straighten their posture and look more in control.
- They get quite emotional once the reality has hit home that they are in control at last!

Take notes;

If you are watching the video download available via www.recoveryfromstroke.co.uk

I hope that you find the contents of the video useful?

Please don't be put off by the simplicity of the content; it is far more effective when simplified; aiming at ones basic language; to stop the person's unconscious mind from getting bored quickly.

Keep it lively energetic and best of all make it fun.

If you have any questions please email me at recoveryfromstroke@gmail.com

I have been studying Hypnosis and the power of the mind since 1974 and have performed many types of therapies on many thousands of people over the years as well as teaching this fascinating subject.

Because I purposely steer away from using technical jargon when either teaching or performing therapies, does not make the power of *Shak Therapy* any less effective.

Through experience the more basic the language the more effective *Shak Therapy* is! I.e. if you talk in the manner of 123 / ABC you will get results, if you talk 1234 / ABCD then it's too drawn out and complicated.

Keep it simple; fun and energetic, But! Not too much that it appears to take away from the client the seriousness of their condition!

It is a case of not crossing the line.

And now; we will talk about the metaphor.

The Metaphor to suit your own location!

Follow this script when inputting the metaphor used for making Shak Therapy more effective!

Fill in the Blank spaces provided for you; using locations from your unique geographical area! In order that the person receiving Shak Therapy understands their own location to make it work better!

Below is the Metaphor used for Areas where I; "John W. Green" Shak Therapy Founder lives?

The Metaphor:

I would like you to use your fantastic imagination and imagine that you are on the telephone talking to

Your friend lives in _Leeds___ you are here in ____Hull____ chatting on the Telephone to your friend in ___Leeds____ and the telephone conversation is going from you to your friend via __Pontefract____ telephone exchange! You are chatting ok to your friend from your home in ____Hull____ to ___Leeds_____ via _Pontefract___ when all of a sudden… __Pontefract____ telephone exchange explodes… It just blows up and disappears…BUT! In a mille-second you are instantly diverted to _Scunthorpe_ Telephone Company and you don't even know that_ Pontefract__ Exchange has blown up! You are diverted to _Scunthorpe__ and your conversation with Your friend is not interrupted at all. You have no idea that _Pontefract__ has had an Explosion because the signal was instantly diverted to your friend via a different way! Clearly and smoothly without any conscious thought! Now that your mind understands this, it is already finding new neuro pathways around the damaged area of your brain.

Continue with: Now that your subconscious or unconscious mind understands the speed at which these signals "are" being diverted it makes it easier to allow these wonderful signals to simply find a new direction, making it easier to re-connect the signals from those once detached feelings from limbs and speech and "**at last**" allowing these lovely feelings to flow to where ever they are needed without any conscious thought getting in the way…

Follow with: You don't need to know **how** it works or **why** it works… You just need to know that it does!

Continue with the Shak Therapy as described in this book (or if you opt to buy the accompanying video download) using touch etc…

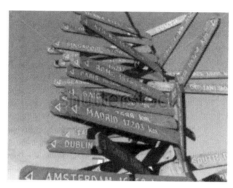

The Metaphor to suit your own location!

Follow this script when inputting the metaphor used for making Shak Therapy more effective!

Fill in the Blank spaces with this script provided for you; using locations from your unique geographical area! In order that the person receiving Shak Therapy understands their own location to make it work better!

Below is the Metaphor for you to <u>**fill in the blank spaces**</u> with your own unique geographical locations:

I would like you to use your fantastic imagination and imagine that you are on the telephone talking to your friend who lives in _____ you are here in _____ chatting on the Telephone to your friend in _____ and the telephone conversation is going from you to your friend via _____ telephone exchange! You are chatting ok to your friend from your home in

_____ to _____ via _____ _
when all of a sudden... _____ telephone exchange explodes... It just blows up and disappears...BUT! In a mille-second you are instantly diverted to _____ Telephone Company; **you don't even know** that _____ Exchange has blown up! You are diverted to _____ and your conversation with your friend is not interrupted at all. You have no idea that _____ has had an Explosion because the signal was instantly diverted to your friend via a different way! Clearly and smoothly without any thought! Now that your mind understands this; it is already finding new ways around the damaged area of your brain.

Continue with:

Now that your subconscious or unconscious mind understands the speed at which these signals "are" being diverted it makes it easier to allow these wonderful signals to simply find a new direction, making it easier to re-connect the signals from those once detached feelings from limbs and speech and "<u>at last</u>" allowing these lovely feelings to flow to where ever they are needed without any conscious thought getting in the way...

Follow with: You don't need to know **how** it works or **why** it works... You just need to know that it does!

Continue with the Shak Therapy as described in this book or if you opt to buy the accompanying video download using touch etc...

Add humour to your initial meeting.

It is very important to note that; when you first meet a client; you inject a sense of confident, jolliness, bubbly chat and humour! This will stimulate the client's subconscious and immediately divert their thoughts away from feeling down and depressed. It will also make them more interested in you as a person. Especially as you are the one that has just made them put on the kettle if the client is able! (For instance) plenty of smiles from you, will show confidence in your own abilities and put away the initial doubt that just about every person has when they are about to have 'Shak therapy' for the very first time.

Speak metaphorically

Supplied with the video download (available www.recoveryfromstroke.co.uk) and in this booklet, is the exact metaphor that has helped quite literally hundreds of people to get around a damaged part of their brain to aid in their healing process, with some people this metaphor will instantly work! Dependent upon the extent of their brain damage (along with aphasia) and with others there will be some improvement (no matter how small, they and their family will see this improvement) from then on any improvement can be improved upon again and again.

TOUCH

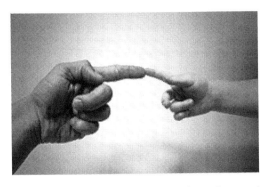

The next phase; once the metaphor has been implanted; is touch to stimulate the mind into being even more curious and wanting to send feeling thoughts to exactly where you are touching! Making their mind work so fast and now; at last being able to divert the thoughts around any damaged areas of the brain to follow where you are touching along with fast excited talking and actually making the mind become more in contact with the limbs! Effectively you are making the persons limbs be a part of their unconscious movements (reflex movements)… this doubled up with visually seeing what is happening to themselves is mind blowing and so stimulating, all the person can now do; is listen to you and believe in you so much that their own depression is floating away; taking away their negative mental blockages and allowing a new way of thinking to take place which causes them to feel alive and determined and allowing these amazing feelings to flow.

You as the therapist will feel pretty drained whilst performing Shak Therapy™ because you will really be caught up in the moment (with practice) hence a nice cup of tea to keep your mouth moist whilst working with your client.

You will get faster and more excited as you are watching the changes take place right before your very eyes.

(Remember every person is different and some changes may not be as big or as fast as others)

Improvement is what we are looking for!

Finish your tea and consolidate

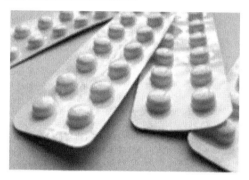

Always emphasise the importance of **never stopping medication without their Doctors advice!** This is very important with any type of therapy you may do on a person when using holistic methods!

Medicine and holistic methods do work hand in hand when circumstances allow.

SHAK

THERAPY

Shak Therapy.

Developed and fine tuned in to what it is today! Shak Therapy has been used on countless numbers of people with very impressive results; Ranging from what can only be described as miraculous to a definite improvement, Able to be improved upon even move!

Shak Therapy is not the miracle cure! Yet! It is a very powerful tool that can aid in the revitalisation of once immobile limbs, Ranging from stroke survivors to accident survivors!

The word Shak is a Latin word which means "To Remedy" and that is what it does to help many people, it literally instils (revitalises) feelings and movement to what where once lifeless or very clumsy limbs and balances out thought patterns, it balances out a person mind very quickly and once lost; cognitive abilities come flooding back exponentially in many cases!

Shak has without any doubt what so ever! Instantly brought speech back to stroke survivors that have lost the ability to speak! Shak has shocked the receiver by the mere fact that they suddenly regained feelings in their tongue and clarity of mind follows virtually instantly.

So let us recap:

1. Add humour to your initial meeting i.e. what letter comes after "s" in the alphabet etc.
2. Speak metaphorically (instil the metaphor for this particular condition)
3. Touch matched with fast excited chat to stimulate the subconscious even more. Use words like Magic, fantastic, brilliant, amazing etc.
4. Finish your tea and consolidate (never stop medication till your doctor says etc...) and leave!
5. Ask the client to describe how they are feeling?
6. Ask the client to move limbs / Talk / read lines from a book.
7. Ask client to touch their fingers to their thumb etc.

Useful links:

www.Recoveryfromstroke.co.uk

www.shak-therapy.com

Email: recoveryfromstroke@gmal.com

Made in the USA
Lexington, KY
04 September 2019